In Control

help with incontinence

PENNY MARES

GW00690301

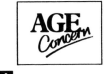

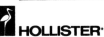

Age Concern would like to acknowledge the generous financial sponsorship provided by Hollister Ltd to allow this book to reach a wider audience than would otherwise have been possible.
A summary of Hollister's products and services begins on page 85

Published by Age Concern England
Astral House
1268 London Road
London SW16 4EJ

Editor   Lee Bennett
Design   Eugenie Dodd
Production   Joyce O'Shaughnessy
Printed by Grosvenor Press, Portsmouth

British Library Cataloguing in Publication Data
Mares, Penny
  In Control
  1.Old Persons. Incontinency
  1. Title ll. Age Concern England
  616.63

ISBN 0-86242-088-1

Cover photograph by Sunil Gupta

Drawings on pages 33, 36-37, 64 by Robin Dodd
and on pages 14-15, 22-23, 49, 51, 54 by Maurizia Merati

Contents

Foreword

It is now estimated that somewhere between 2 and 3 million people in the United Kingdom suffer from incontinence, a large percentage of these being over the age of 65. Incontinence, however, is not inevitable as we get older; and over the last five years more and more sources of help have been made available.

Hollister Limited are delighted to sponsor this excellent new publication which looks at many of the common problems associated with incontinence and how to obtain advice and support. I am sure that this book will be of tremendous interest and benefit to all concerned.

Patrick Baker
Vice President/General Manager
Hollister Limited, United Kingdom

About the Author

Penny Mares is a consultant in health education and training. She has been researching and writing handbooks and training resources for professionals and the public for over ten years. She is currently a member of the Open College Health Courses Team.

Acknowledgements

Penny Mares would like to thank Niccy Whitaker and Mary Tidyman for their contribution in researching and drafting sections of the material for this handbook. Niccy Whitaker is a lecturer in adult education, freelance writer and co-author of several books and training resources on aspects of health and caring. Mary Tidyman currently works for the Health Education Authority and was involved with the Health in Old Age Programme; she is co-author of a number of health education publications.

Thanks also to the following people who contributed ideas and information for this handbook: Barbara Hamilton, an independent continence and training adviser; Barbara Meredith, Evelyn McEwen and Sally West of Age Concern England; Dee Hemsley; June Thompson; Helen White and colleagues at the Dene Centre Continence Advisory Service, Newcastle upon Tyne; Margaret Brotherton; the continence advisers at St Pancras Hospital, London; Jenny Clarkin, Marilyn Hepworth and other members and friends of Garforth Carers Group; and all those who talked to us about their own feelings and experience of living with incontinence.

Introduction

This book provides information about the choices that may be available to you whether you suffer from incontinence or look after someone who does. As an older person suffering from this problem, you may live alone or with someone else or in a residential or nursing home or a hospital.

Wherever you live, you (and those who care for you) need to know as much as possible about incontinence and how to cure or cope with it. This book will help you decide what you need and how to go about getting it.

Remember you are not alone if you suffer from this condition. There are likely to be many other people in your town or village — perhaps in your own street — who have been able to regain control over incontinence, and over their lives, by getting the right help.

What is Incontinence?

Incontinence — loss of control over the bladder or the bowel — is a problem which affects people of all ages. In Britain an estimated one in twenty people suffer from loss of continence at some point in their lives.

Although older people are more likely to experience incontinence than younger people, it is not an inevitable part of ageing. Two out of three people over the age of 85 have no problem. With present medical knowledge, doctors estimate that one in every two incontinence problems can be cured. If a condition cannot be cured completely, it can always be improved with professional help, so that the person affected, like the woman whose experience is described below, can control the incontinence and lead a more normal life.

Peggy The first doctor she saw told Peggy that she'd just have to put up with a bit of leaking as she got older. But it was really getting her down, so she asked another GP at the health centre who was very good — she did tests, and the nurse helped Peggy sort out a routine so that she could cope with her leaky waterworks without worrying all the time. The second doctor had said to her, 'Don't let anyone tell you it's something you just have to put up with at your age, because it isn't true'.

Incontinence is not a disease in itself. It is a sign that something else is wrong, and it can have many different causes. Some of these are explained in the chapters 'Understanding Urinary Incontinence' and 'Understanding Faecal Incontinence'.

Deciding to seek help

It is important to get help early so that incontinence can be investigated to find out the cause, and steps taken to control it.

Many people do not get help early because they feel ashamed or embarrassed to talk about it. Incontinence is a subject that we don't talk about in public, perhaps because from our earliest childhood we are taught that having accidents, or losing control over when we go to the toilet, is wrong and shameful. Yet when we started writing this book we were surprised at the number of people who showed an interest and who told us about their own problems, or about the experiences of friends or relatives. Many felt that the difficult part was making the decision to seek help. Most found that health professionals were easier to talk to and more understanding than they had expected.

Becoming incontinent makes many people feel less confident in themselves so that it is harder to ask for help. If you are affected by incontinence, you may be doubtful that there really are ways of improving your condition and making your life more comfortable.

The experiences of John, Emily and Joan described in the next few pages show how three people with different kinds of incontinence found help. We hope their experiences will encourage you to feel confident about seeking professional help as early as possible. If you do not feel you can do this yourself, perhaps there is someone close to you, possibly a relative or a carer, who could do it for you.

John John, aged 72, lives with his wife, Edith, in a house with the toilet on the first floor. John has difficulty getting about and can only walk with the help of a Zimmer frame. They are a happy couple, with friends who visit regularly. Their son comes once a month and takes them out for a drive or a meal.

John finds it hard to get upstairs to the toilet. He keeps a covered bucket in the hall which he uses when he needs to urinate. Recently he has found it more difficult to reach the bucket in time. He began to dread having visitors or going out because he was afraid he might wet himself in front of other people. Though she sympathised, Edith became rather depressed at not going out or seeing friends any more. She mentioned the situation to her GP who arranged to examine John and test his urine to make sure that the incontinence was not caused by a problem needing treatment, such as an enlarged prostate gland or a urine infection. As the doctor found no obvious cause, he suggested that the continence adviser might be able to help and arranged for her to visit.

John felt quite embarrassed at the idea of talking to a stranger about such a private matter, which he thought was probably an inevitable part of getting old, but he found the continence adviser was friendly and sympathetic. She asked John when the problem had started, how many times he passed water during the day, whether he had to hurry to reach the toilet, and other details so that she could assess what help would be most appropriate.

The continence adviser suggested a sheath system for collecting urine which John could wear when visitors came or when he was going out, so that he need no longer worry about having an accident. This is a light weight device, attached to the body with adhesive, which collects the urine and is quite comfortable to wear (see drawing on page 51). Each sheath is worn for up to one or two days, but they are available through the GP on prescription so that cost is not a problem.

After showing John and Edith how to use the sheath system, the continence adviser asked them to try it out for a few days to make sure they were happy with it. She also offered to arrange for the loan of a commode for use in the hall, if they preferred that to the covered bucket.

At first John felt a bit awkward because Edith has to help him use the sheath system, but she says she doesn't mind a bit and is very pleased that she can do something to help him lead a more normal life again. He says he feels a huge sense of relief at knowing he can now manage without dreading an embarrassing accident any more.

Joan Joan is a widow in her early sixties with four grown up children. For many years she has had problems of leaking urine, particularly when she laughs or coughs or exerts herself. This condition was gradually getting worse, to the point where she needed to change her pants several times a day to be comfortable and avoid the risk of smelling. She usually wore a couple of sanitary pads if she went out.

Joan finally decided she needed some help, but was rather embarrassed about discussing her plight with the GP, as she did not feel he would be sympathetic. Instead, she mentioned it to the practice nurse at the health centre and was surprised at how ready the nurse was to listen and try to help. Joan answered the nurse's questions about when the leaking had started (after her second child was born), how often and when it occurred, and how much leakage there was.

The nurse explained that Joan had stress incontinence and that it would almost certainly improve if she practiced some exercises to strengthen her pelvic floor muscles. She explained how to do pelvic floor exercises and gave Joan a written sheet about them. The exercises were not difficult, and Joan was so determined to improve control over her bladder that she practised them several times each day while she was busy with other things — watching TV, washing up, or waiting at the bus stop. She was delighted that in just a few weeks she began to notice a real improvement in her condition. She now says she wishes she had got help sooner.

Emily Emily is 84 years old and suffers from confusion. She has recently moved into a residential home because her daughter no longer feels able to cope with looking after her. Emily is confused about where she is, and wanders a lot.

When she was living with her daughter, she was more or less

continent during the day, but used to wet her bed several times at night, leading to disturbed sleep for herself and her daughter. After moving into the residential home, Emily started wetting herself during the day as well as at night, though she usually asked for the toilet if she needed to open her bowels.

The initial response of staff in the home was to use pads and pants during the day and night, in order to avoid the nuisance caused by Emily repeatedly wetting herself. Emily's daughter felt concerned that daytime continence had got so much worse, and asked the staff whether something more could be done.

The continence adviser for the area was invited in to make an assessment and suggest ways of managing the problem. By talking to Emily's daughter and the staff of the home, she was able to assess Emily's general condition, and how and when her continence problems developed. She established that Emily's apparent incontinence was not caused by a loss of bladder control, but by her confusion. Moving into a new environment had temporarily made Emily more confused and less able to cope with routine tasks like remembering to go to the toilet.

The continence adviser suggested that the staff could try to establish a regular toilet routine for Emily, so that she was reminded and taken to the lavatory at regular times throughout the day. This quickly led to improved control over when she emptied her bladder, with only occasional accidents. Emily's last drink of the day is now given a little earlier than before and she is taken to the toilet at bedtime. She wears pads and pants only during the night so that her sleep is not disturbed.

Deciding what you need

It is never too late to do something about incontinence, but the longer it is left, the greater the risk of further complications. If you feel reluctant to admit to yourself that you have a bowel or bladder condition or you look after someone who denies that there is a problem, it may help to read the suggestions on pages 27-29.

Understanding Urinary Incontinence

If you or someone you love or care for has a bladder problem, this chapter may help you to understand the causes. The first part explains how the bladder works. The second part looks at the symptoms and the common causes of urinary incontinence.

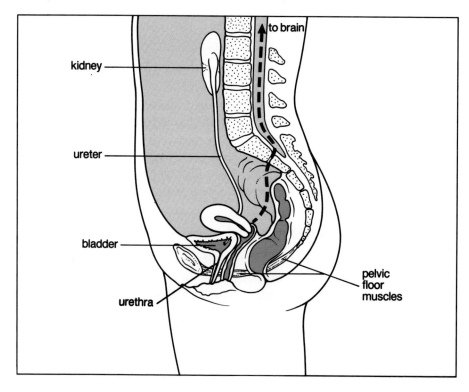

How the urinary system works

From early childhood we learn to control when and where we empty our bladder. This control is achieved by the urinary system — a combined effort of the kidneys, bladder and brain, as shown in the drawings on these two pages.

The bladder in most adults can hold about one pint of urine, sometimes less in older people. As the bladder fills, it sends messages along the nerves to the brain. When this happens, you become aware that you need to pass urine. At an appropriate moment, the brain sends a message to the bladder muscles to contract, and the urine is pushed through the urethra.

Most people empty their bladders four to six times a day, but with age they may need to do this more frequently. Emotions can also affect the messages from the brain, which is why excitement, fear or worry may make you want to empty your bladder more often.

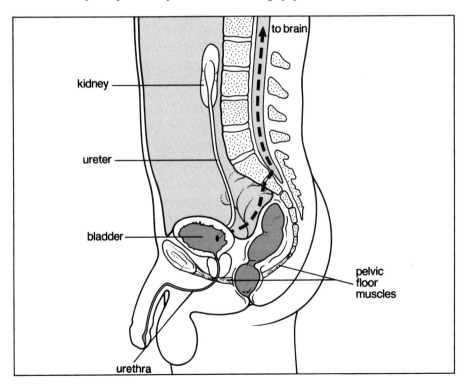

Common incontinence problems

This section describes five common types of urinary incontinence and the symptoms associated with them. Possible treatments are briefly described, but there is more information about different kinds of treatment in the chapter 'Regaining Control'.

Urgency or urge incontinence

You may notice that:

▶ you need to go to the lavatory frequently (more than about six times in the day and once during the night);

▶ you have to rush to get to the toilet in time, with or without leaking before you get there;

▶ your bed is sometimes damp at night.

Why does it happen? The bladder muscles start to contract against your will before the bladder is full. This can make you want to pass water more frequently, or more urgently, than normal. Urgency — needing to rush to the toilet, but without leakage — is a signal that something is wrong. Urge incontinence is the term used when there is leakage as well.

Who does it affect? Urgency is one of the commonest bladder problems among older men and women. Sometimes there is no obvious cause. Sometimes it is caused by a condition which affects the brain or the nerves controlling messages going to and from the bladder (for example, a stroke, Parkinson's disease, dementia, multiple sclerosis or diabetes).

Can it be treated? Urgency and urge incontinence can usually be treated quite easily by a combination of medicines and bladder retraining.

Overflow incontinence

You may notice that:

▶ you want to go the lavatory more often;

▶ you have to strain to pass urine;

▶ your water comes out as a trickle rather than a stream;

▶ you have to rush to get to the toilet in time, sometimes leaking before you get there;

▶ you dribble all the time;

▶ your bladder does not feel empty after passing urine.

Why does it happen? There is something preventing the urine in your bladder passing through the urethra to the outside. Sometimes urine builds up in the bladder and the bladder never completely empties, though you may not realise this.

Who does it affect? Overflow incontinence can affect both men and women, though it is more common in men. It is often caused by an enlarged prostate gland, especially in older men. The prostate gland squeezes the urethra so that less urine can pass through it. Sometimes constipation can cause these symptoms. The bowel is next to the bladder; and a very full, constipated bowel may squeeze against the urethra, as shown in the drawings on pages 22-23. Sometimes a serious illness may affect the brain's control over the bladder.

Can it be treated? Treatment will depend on the cause. An enlarged prostate gland may need a simple operation. Constipation can usually be treated and cured quite easily.

Stress incontinence

You may notice that:

▶ your bladder leaks when you laugh, cough, or make some physical effort like lifting or jogging.

Why does it happen? Stress incontinence is caused by stress or pressure on weakened muscles — it is not due to emotional stress. The muscles that surround and support your bladder, rather like a hammock, are called the pelvic floor muscles. They may become weakened so they can no longer support and close the bladder and urethra as efficiently. Urine leaks out when there is a sudden pressure on these muscles. This often starts as a slight problem, but it can get worse over time if it is not treated.

Who does it affect? This mainly affects women and is common during pregnancy or after childbirth when the pelvic floor muscles may be stretched. It also affects older women after the change of life. This is because changes in the hormone levels in your body after the menopause can affect the efficient working of the muscles supporting your bladder. Hormone changes can also cause the urethra to become drier and less elastic, making it more difficult to close tightly.

Can it be treated? Stress incontinence can often be prevented or completely cured by simple exercises over several months to strengthen the pelvic floor muscles (see page 40).

Underactive bladder

You may notice that:

▶ you have to strain to empty your bladder;

▶ you have to press your abdomen (tummy) to get the urine out;

▶ you sometimes dribble;

▶ you need to go to the lavatory often.

Why does it happen? The bladder muscles are not able to contract properly to squeeze the urine out through the urethra to the outside. A large volume of urine can build up in the bladder — sometimes reaching as much as four pints.

Who does it affect? This problem can affect both men and women. It is common among people suffering from diabetes, which may damage the nerves in the bladder so that they cannot signal to the brain when the bladder is full. Diabetes can develop as you get older, and an underactive bladder is sometimes the first noticeable sign of it. An injury to the lower part of the spinal cord can also cause this problem.

Can it be treated? A very thin catheter can be inserted every so often to empty the bladder when it becomes full. This may sound alarming, but most people learn to use their own catheter quite easily and enjoy the greater freedom it gives them.

Dribbling

You may notice that:

▶ you dribble urine after you've been to the toilet and passed water.

Why does it happen? Some urine remains in the urethra after you pass water and then leaks out later. Normally the muscles in the urethra expel this urine, but they may become weaker in older people.

Who does it affect? This is most common in men, as the urethra is much longer than in women. A man who has had his prostate gland removed (see page 45) may experience greater problems, as there may be a cavity where the prostate was, which can fill with urine. Women are sometimes affected by dribbling, but usually to a lesser degree.

Can it be treated? Many women find it helps to sit over the toilet for a few moments longer once the flow of urine has stopped, before wiping with toilet paper.

Men may find it helps after passing water to run a finger firmly forward from back to front along the urethra — this is the narrow tube that can be felt behind the scrotum. Repeat this until no more urine dribbles from the penis. (Shaking the penis does not help, as the urine is usually trapped further back in the urethra.)

Other possible causes of incontinence

There are other factors which may cause or add to loss of bladder control. These too can often be cured or improved. If you look after someone suffering from incontinence, you can seek help together. More information about treatment is given in the chapter 'Regaining Control'.

Constipation

This is a common cause of urinary incontinence in older people. But is is not inevitable, and can often be treated and cleared up quite easily.

Infection in the urinary system

This can result in a loss of bladder control which may clear up when the infection is diagnosed and treated.

Difficulty in getting to the toilet

If you are confined to bed or cannot move about very quickly, or if you're slow at getting dressed or undressed, you may sometimes wet yourself because you cannot reach the toilet in time. This is not true incontinence — your urinary system is still working properly, but your circumstances are slowing you down.

You can get specialist help to arrange your routine and your surroundings to make daily tasks as easy as possible for you or the person caring for you. Sometimes small changes can make all the difference (for example, changing the way the door opens or putting handrails in the toilet, or moving the bed so the commode is easy to get to).

Medicines (drugs)

Taking certain medicines or drugs, such as tranquillisers, 'water tablets' (diuretics) and some medicines used for chronic bronchitis and asthma may increase the urge to pass water. Sleeping tablets, alcohol and some medicines used for arthritis can dull the sensations so that when the bladder becomes full, you are not able to feel the urge to pass water. Your doctor may be able to help by changing the dose, or the type of medicine you take.

Emotional upsets

These can affect the way in which the brain controls the emptying of your bladder. Excitement, fear or worry may make you want to empty your bladder more often. Practising the simple relaxation exercise in 'Regaining Control' on page 38 can reduce anxiety and may help you get a better night's sleep.

Confusion

If you are looking after someone who is severely confused (with dementia or because of a serious medical condition), there may be incontinence problems because the person forgets to go to or cannot find the toilet, or has difficulties undoing clothing. It is helpful to remind them or take them to the toilet regularly, and make sure clothes are easy to remove.

Changes in surroundings

Moving to a new home, or going into hospital or a residential home is a major emotional upheaval which also upsets the the normal daily routine. It means getting used to a new environment, making friends with new faces and learning a brand new routine. Just getting familiar with where the new toilets are can take time. It's not surprising or unusual for someone to go through a phase of incontinence after this kind of upheaval. If you are caring for someone in these circumstances, try to give as much reassurance as you can. If you become anxious, you will only increase the stress on the person you care for.

With sympathetic care and help, many people find that the problems disappear as they settle in and get to know their new surroundings. Don't panic over one or two accidents.

What can be done?

Turn to 'Getting Help' for more information about who you can go to for advice, what kind of questions you'll be asked, and what is likely to happen if your problem needs investigating.

Understanding Faecal Incontinence

This chapter looks at the symptoms and common causes of faecal incontinence (pronounced 'fee-kal'). Loss of control over the bowels is less common than urinary incontinence, but it can be very distressing for those who suffer from it and those who care for them. Like urinary incontinence, faecal incontinence can always be improved and often cured.

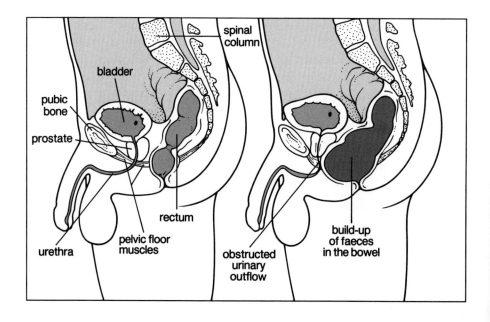

Your bowels and the digestive system

Food taken into the mouth passes down into the stomach where digestion begins. From the stomach food passes along a series of tubes called the small and large intestines and then into the bowel. Just as the bladder stores and pumps out urine, the bowel stores and pumps out faeces (see the drawings on these two pages). It is normally kept closed by a thick ring of muscle called the sphincter. When the rectum begins to fill up, you feel the urge to open your bowels. Messages are sent along the nerves to your brain and then back to the sphincter and rectum, to pump out the faeces through the back passage (or anus).

Common bowel problems

This section describes some common bowel problems and what can be done to help them.

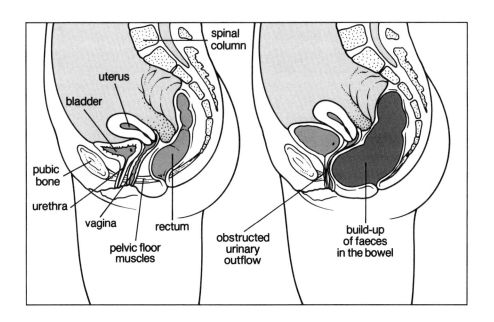

Anxiety about constipation

Many older people worry about getting constipated, but not everyone opens their bowels every day. Anything from three times a day to twice a week is perfectly normal. If you have a small appetite, you may not be eating enough to warrant a daily bowel movement. If you feel healthy otherwise, and you do not suffer from hard faeces or have to strain, you should not worry if you do not open your bowels every day.

Using laxatives daily

It is important not to take laxatives without your doctor's advice. In the past, laxatives were thought to help keep the bowels regular and healthy, but today doctors do not advise regular use. It is thought that laxatives can increase the chances of constipation because they make the bowel muscles lazy — they come to depend on the laxative to work properly.

Constipation

Constipation, or straining to open the bowels and passing hard faeces, is a common condition among older people, but it is not inevitable. Changes in diet, an increase in the amount you drink, and regular movement or exercise — if these are possible — may help the problem (see also 'Regaining Control'). Sometimes diarrhoea can also result from serious constipation.

Diarrhoea or leaking

This can be caused by an upset stomach or 'tummy bug'. It can also happen if you become very constipated. This is because watery faeces begin to leak around the hard faeces in the bowel. Someone who has diarrhoea is more likely to develop leaking and loss of bowel control. Diarrhoea should normally disappear once the upset stomach or constipation is treated.

Alternating constipation and diarrhoea

This may be a sign that there is a disease of the intestine or rectum, and it is important to see your doctor for help. Treatment will depend on the cause.

Changes in normal bowel habits

If your normal pattern changes unexpectedly — for example, if you find you are opening your bowels much more or much less often than usual — and if there is no obvious reason, such as a change in the food you are eating or the amount of exercise you're getting, then you should tell your doctor.

Blood in the faeces

You may notice blood when you open your bowel. This can be caused by piles, which can sometimes bleed when faeces are passed, or by bleeding from the intestine or rectum. If you are worried about this, you should see your doctor.

Black faeces

If you are taking iron tablets, this will make your faeces look a darker colour than usual. Black faeces can also be a sign of bleeding from the stomach or intestine, and you should see your doctor.

Common causes of faecal incontinence

Leaking may be caused by weakening of the sphincter which keeps the rectum closed while faeces are stored. This can be the result of lack of exercise, childbirth, or straining to pass hard faeces.

Injury or damage to the spine or brain (for example, from an accident or stroke) may affect the nerves that pass messages between the rectum and brain. Your brain may have lost control over the messages which tell your rectum when to empty.

Other things that can make faecal incontinence more likely are:

▶ being confined to bed;

▶ being unable to move about quickly;

▶ being slow at dressing or undressing;

▶ taking certain medicines (such as pain killers containing codeine) — some drugs can cause or increase constipation leading to leaking of watery faeces.

- ▶ depression;
- ▶ emotional upsets;
- ▶ reducing the amount that you normally eat or drink.

What can be done?

If you are worried about any of the problems we have described — especially constipation, a change in your normal bowel habits, blood in your faeces, incontinence or leaking — it is important to get help from your GP or a community nurse, so that the cause can be found. The condition can be cured or improved with the right treatment.

Do not ignore these symptoms, or try to treat yourself with laxatives without taking advice from the community nurse and/or your GP. One solution for immobile people who are constipated is the use of suppositories or an enema given once a week by the community nurse.

Read 'Getting Help' if you would like more information about who you can go to for advice, what kind of questions you'll be asked, and what is likely to happen if your problem needs investigating.

Getting Help

People who suffer from incontinence often feel cut off from others because they cannot talk about it and they somehow feel that it is up to them to cope on their own. Yet coming to terms with these difficult feelings and finding the right person to talk to can be the first step towards a more comfortable and fuller life. Equally, someone caring for a person with incontinence should seek help so that coping with the problem becomes as manageable as possible.

This chapter explores some of the reasons behind these awkward feelings, and suggests ways of talking about incontinence and how to find the right person to talk to. It also gives you information about the questions you may be asked and how to be prepared for them.

Talking about incontinence

Many people find it embarrassing to talk about incontinence. This is perhaps because we are taught from an early age that emptying our bladder and bowels are private activities, and many of us may have been taught that these body functions are also somehow dirty or shameful. Some people find it hard to accept that there is a problem, let alone to ask for help with something that seems so personal and private. These feelings are understandable but it is important to try and overcome them, and find the confidence to talk to someone. Some people find it easier to start by talking to a sympathetic relative or close friend. Others find it easier to talk in confidence to a doctor or nurse.

You may be worried about how to describe your problems. You may feel unfamiliar with the medical terms used by doctors and nurses when they talk about the intimate parts of your body and its functions. You may wonder what words or phrases you should use when talking about your condition. Health care professionals are used to talking to people who describe their problems in widely differing ways, and they are unlikely to be surprised by any terms which you use. Simply talk about what is wrong in the language which you feel most comfortable with.

Caring for someone with incontinence

It is not unusual for someone who has become incontinent to find this difficult to accept or acknowledge. People who depend on someone else to care for them may deny or try to hide the fact that they have a problem, for a variety of reasons. They may find incontinence and the loss of dignity that comes with it too painful or embarrassing to face. They may be frightened that a breakdown in such a basic body function means they are seriously ill, or perhaps dying. They may fear that those who care for them will no longer want to look after them, or will stop loving them. If they live in a residential home, they may be afraid of being asked to leave.

The experiences of the caring relatives outlined below illustrate some of the feelings you may have had.

Nelson 'I think Dad had convinced himself they'd throw him out of the Home so he just pretended it wasn't happening and denied it even when he'd obviously wet himself. That's what exasperated the staff — not the actual mopping up. But the Home is well run — they arranged for someone to assess his condition and in the end we got him to use a sheath system, but he still says things like, "I don't know what I've got to wear all this paraphernalia for". I suppose it's his way of coping — he just can't face up to the embarrassment.'

Ella 'I felt it was the last straw when I realised my mother was beginning to suffer from faecal incontinence. I thought, "that's it...I can't take any more". Then I suppose I began to come to terms with it, and I kept telling myself it's just the same as cleaning up the kids when they were babies — that never bothered me. Of course, it's not the same when it's your mother, but it helped to hang on to that thought. I think she probably finds it quite humiliating, knowing the woman she was. I try to show her that it doesn't affect how I feel about her as a person. We cope, but neither of us finds it easy.'

Dorothy 'My mother-in-law lives with us and I began to realise she was wetting herself now and then — I'd find smelly things in the laundry basket; but she never said anything to either of us. Ken wouldn't talk to her about it because he was too embarrassed. I actually phoned one of the continence helplines, because I just didn't know what to say to Ken's mum. The adviser was very reassuring and suggested I should just ask her, "Are you finding you sometimes don't make it to the toilet in time?". I think when she realised I wasn't going to accuse her or criticise her for it, she actually seemed relieved to be able to talk about it. I think she was quite frightened about what was happening to her body, as well as being painfully embarrassed.'

Finding out what's wrong

The way your problem will be treated and the chances of curing it depend on finding out the cause. There may be one cause or a number of factors which a trained professional will be able to discover after asking you some questions and, in some cases, carrying out a physical examination. They may also do some simple tests, such as examining a sample of your urine or faeces. If they think that the causes of your problem need looking into further, you may be referred to a hospital consultant.

Who can help?

There may be several health professionals who could help, depending on your circumstances and the part of the country where you live. The professional you are most likely to make first contact with is the:

▶ general practitioner

▶ community/district nurse

▶ health visitor

▶ continence adviser

General practitioner May be involved with your treatment and the management of your condition even if you go to another health adviser first. The GP may want to refer you to a specialist for further investigations. If you need certain types of equipment, you may be able to get these on prescription from the doctor.

Community nurse or health visitor In some areas of the country they give advice or practical help with incontinence problems. You can phone your doctor's surgery or health centre and ask to speak to either of them.

Continence adviser A specialist nurse, trained and experienced in dealing with continence problems. Sometimes continence advisers run clinics at local health centres as well as visiting people at home. They may also be able to visit someone in a residential or nursing home, though this varies from area to area. Your GP surgery, local clinic or health centre will be able to tell you how to contact the continence adviser for your area — if there is one. From the end of 1991, continence advisers rather than GPs will also prescribe products and devices for incontinence.

If you have any difficulty in getting in touch with a continence adviser, the Association of Continence Advisors or the local Age Concern may be able to help you find one (see 'Helpful Organisations' on page 68).

The important thing is to find someone to talk to who makes you feel comfortable. If the first person you ask is not very helpful, don't be discouraged. One older woman who found her GP was rather unsympathetic went instead to see the district nurse, who was able to arrange for a continence adviser to visit her and make an assessment.

If you feel you would like more information about incontinence before you see a health professional, you may like to use one of the confidential advice services or telephone helplines listed in 'Resources and Information'.

Other professionals who may also be able to offer different kinds of help or support are:

▶ social worker

▶ occupational therapist

▶ physiotherapist

▶ obstetric physiotherapist

You will find more information about how these people can help on pages 55-56.

What your health adviser will want to know

To assess your problem, the doctor or nurse you see (your 'health adviser') will ask a few simple questions about your bladder or bowel control. They will also want to know about your general health and whether you are taking any medicines. They may ask you about your home circumstances or visit you to find out whether there are reasons which make it difficult for you to get to the toilet in time. As a carer looking after someone with incontinence, you may need to assist with giving information.

The questions about bladder or bowel control will vary according to each person's problem, but we have listed some of the more usual on page 32. You can help the health adviser by being prepared with the answers to these questions.

The questions are listed separately for bladder and bowel problems. (You may be asked questions about both bowels and your bladder, as something wrong with one system can often affect the other.) Be sure to mention any other symptoms you have which may be worrying you if you are not asked about them.

Questions about bladder problems

If you have urinary incontinence, these are some of the questions you may be asked:

How many times do you pass water each day?

Do you ever not make it to the toilet in time?

Do you leak when you cough, laugh or run?

Do you have any trouble actually passing water?

Do you ever dribble after you have passed water?

Is the bed ever wet in the morning?

Questions about bowel problems

These are some of the questions you may be asked if you have trouble controlling your bowels:

Do you have to get up to open your bowels at night?

Do you suffer from constipation/or hard faeces?

Do you take laxatives?

Do you suffer from diarrhoea?

Do you ever not make it to the toilet in time?

Does it ever hurt when you open your bowels?

Do you ever pass blood with your bowel motion?

Keeping a record

You will probably find it easier to answer these questions if you have kept a record of when you empty your bladder or have a bowel movement over a few days. This need not be anything complicated — just a simple chart which shows when you passed water if you have a bladder problem, or when you opened your bowels if you have a bowel problem. Remember to note whether it was in the toilet or not.

RECORD OF PASSING URINE

Day	Time	Place where leaking occurred	Was urine passed into the toilet?
Mon.	8.00am	Leaking along the corridor.	
Mon.	9·00am	No leaking.	Yes
Mon.	10.45am	Leaking while standing at Kitchen sink.	No
Mon.	12.15pm	No leaking	Yes
Mon.	2.30pm	Pants were damp when I got to toilet	Yes

If you record your bowel movements, it is also useful to note the consistency of the bowel motion or faeces — was it loose, firm or hard?

RECORD OF BOWEL MOVEMENTS

Day	Time	Place where leaking occurred	Were faeces passed into the toilet?
Mon.	9.30am	Leaked while getting to toilet.	Yes-loose faeces
Wed.	10.00am	Leaked while getting out of chair	Yes-loose faeces
Thur.	7.15pm	No leaking	Yes-firm, normal
Fri.	6.00pm	Leaked while getting out of bed.	Yes-watery

If you prefer, you can make notes in the form of a diary. Here are some points to include if you have a bladder problem:

When you pass water Note the time of day and measure the amount of urine if you can (using a plastic measuring jug to collect your urine is an easy way).

When you are wet Note the time of day and whether you have to change your clothes.

What you drink Note the number of cups or glasses you have in the day. Include everything you drink (eg tea, coffee, juice, soft drinks, beer, wine and water).

Here are some points to include if you have a bowel problem:

When you open your bowels Note the time of day and the consistency of your bowel motion (loose/firm/hard).

When you are continent Note the time of day and whether you have to change your clothes.

What you eat and drink Note all the meals and snacks you have.

What else will your health adviser do?

The person that you see will be able to get a clear picture of your problem by asking questions similar to those outlined in this chapter and from the pattern of passing urine or bowel movements that you record over a few days. They may give you a physical examination and ask for a sample of urine or faeces to test.

Your GP may want to refer you to a hospital consultant for further tests to help discover the cause of your incontinence. These are usually done at an outpatient's clinic. The GP or the hospital staff will explain what the tests are for and how they are done. If you are anxious or have any queries about these investigations, do not hesitate to tell a doctor or nurse what is worrying you — they are there to help and explain.

Regaining Control

This chapter describes the steps you can take to regain control over your bladder or bowels. You may be able to cure the problem completely, or get help to manage it in a way that puts you back in control. There is information about what you can do to help yourself and about some of the common treatments for incontinence.

What can you do for yourself?

It is important to get professional help for incontinence as early as possible, but there is also a lot that you can do yourself to improve your condition and your overall feeling of well-being. If you suffer from mild incontinence, the guidelines in this section may make a noticeable difference and help to prevent your problem getting worse.

A healthy diet

Eating healthily is one of the best things you can do to help yourself. For a balanced diet, eat a variety of foods, keep down the amount of sugar and fat, and eat plenty of fresh fruit, vegetables and cereals. Guidelines on healthy eating now recommend a well-balanced diet high in fibre and bulk to provide all the body needs to function fully. The bulk keeps the bowels working efficiently and helps to prevent constipation.

Serious constipation can cause both bladder and bowel problems so try to establish a regular pattern of bowel movements. Avoid taking laxatives regularly, as it can be more difficult for the bowels to work without them once you stop.

Another reason for eating sensibly is to avoid putting on weight. Carrying extra weight can weaken the pelvic muscles, which may lead to stress incontinence. Being overweight also increases the risk of diabetes and heart disease. Most people tend to put on weight as they get older. Being careful about what you eat and taking some form of exercise, if you can, will help you to avoid becoming overweight.

Getting enough fibre   To make sure that your diet contains enough fibre, you should eat some of the following foods every day: wholemeal bread or chapattis, wholegrain breakfast cereals, lentils or other pulses, bran biscuits, fruit and vegetables.

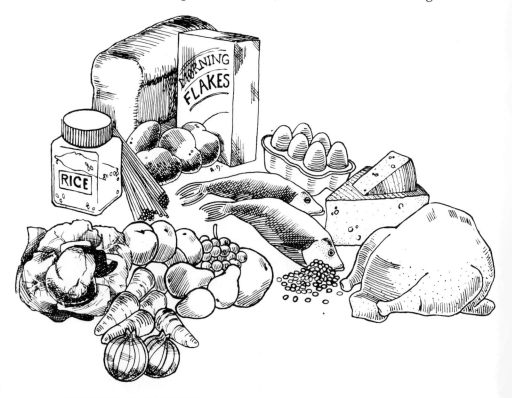

If you are not used to eating foods high in fibre, try making a gradual change in your diet. Drastic changes can cause wind and bowel discomfort. Small changes are worthwhile and easier to stick to. For instance, the first week you might change your breakfast cereal to a high fibre one. The following week, try using bran-based biscuits in place of ones made with white flour, or eating slices of white and wholemeal bread alternately. You can buy bran from wholefood shops and add a spoonful during cooking to pastry, soups, stews and other suitable dishes.

Healthy drinking Many people think they can help their bladder or bowel control by restricting the amount of liquids they drink. In fact the opposite is true — drinking plenty of fluid each day helps the kidneys to function properly and prevents the urine from becoming concentrated. It also helps to prevent constipation. You need between six and nine cups of fluid each day.

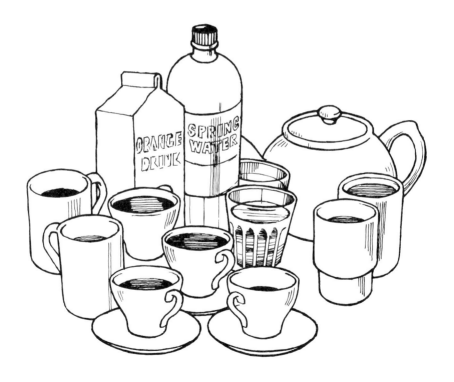

Some people who are incontinent during the night or who need to get up several times to use the toilet find it helps to limit the amount they drink during the evening. Try this for a few days and if it helps, remember to drink plenty of fluid earlier in the day so that you do not reduce the amount you drink overall. If you do not notice any improvement, go back to your normal evening drinking pattern.

People with heart conditions and taking diuretic drugs need to have their fluid intake supervised by the community nurse or GP. It can be dangerous for them to drink too much. They will also need to go to the toilet much more frequently after taking diuretics (see also page 41).

Some drinks, such as tea, coffee, chocolate and alcoholic drinks like beer, produce larger amounts of urine and more quickly than other drinks. Try cutting down on these, and replacing some of them with water, fruit juice, squash, herbal teas or decaffeinated coffee.

Relaxation and exercise

Learning to relax Feeling anxious about your condition can lead to stress and tension. Learning how to relax tense muscles and practising this regularly can reduce stress and help with sleeping problems and depression.

Here is a simple relaxation exercise for you to try:

▶ Find a quiet place. Sit comfortably or lie on your back, and close your eyes.

▶ Begin by tensing your right hand for a moment, then relax it and let it go loose. Continue tensing and relaxing your right arm, moving upward to the shoulder. Repeat the procedure on your right leg, moving up from the foot to the thigh.

▶ Then do the same with the left side of your body. Your arms and legs should feel heavy, relaxed and warm.

▶ Now try relaxing your hip muscles, up through your abdomen to your chest. Let your muscles feel heavy and warm. Concentrate on your breathing and let it slow down.

▶ Let the relaxation flow up into your shoulders, jaw, and face muscles, especially around the eyes and in your forehead.

▶ You will need to practise these steps each day — five minutes will help, or longer if you have the time.

Exercises for general health Try to include some form of gentle exercise in your daily routine. What you can do will depend on your general health and how mobile you are. Any regular movement, however little, is better than nothing. Walking and swimming are both good ways to exercise the whole body.

If you cannot manage these, try doing a few gentle exercises at home. *The Magic of Movement* also published by Age Concern offers a range of gentle exercises especially for older people (see 'Useful Publications' on page 72 for more details). If you have a medical condition or disability which makes movement difficult, check with your doctor first before attempting any exercise.

The important thing is to keep moving if you are able to. This way you will give yourself every chance of overcoming problems of bladder or bowel control that are caused by not being able to get about easily.

Exercises to improve your bladder and bowel control Simple exercises can help tone up the pelvic muscles which are important in controlling bladder and bowels. You can see in the drawings on pages 14-15 how these muscles surround the passages leading from the bladder and bowel.

Women in particular often have weak pelvic muscles. This is sometimes caused by the muscles not returning to their original strength after childbirth. Good control of the pelvic muscles is equally important for men. (These exercises are usually suggested after removal of the prostate gland — see page 45.)

If you suffer from stress incontinence, learning how to control your pelvic muscles and improving their strength may be all you need to become continent. It may be a few weeks before you notice any improvement, so keep doing the exercises a few times a day.

Once you have learned how, you can do them anywhere at any time without anyone knowing. Your health adviser will teach you how to do them.

Exercises for the pelvic muscles You can do these exercises sitting, standing or lying down. Just choose a position you feel relaxed in with your legs slightly apart.

▶ To feel your pelvic floor muscles, imagine that you are trying to control diarrhoea by tightening the muscles around the back passage. These are the muscles which form the back part of the pelvic floor.

▶ Imagine that you are trying to stop passing urine by tightening the muscles around the outlet from the bladder. These muscles make up the front of the pelvic floor. Now relax your muscles.

▶ Then slowly tighten the muscles of your pelvic floor, working from the back to the front while you count to four slowly. Gently let go. Repeat this exercise four times; but do not try more than four contractions each time, as the muscles become too tired to work properly.

▶ When doing the exercises, try not to let the muscles of your thighs, buttocks and abdomen tighten up as well, and keep your breathing even and relaxed.

▶ Once you have got used to these exercises, you should do them at least four times a day — every hour if you can. There is no need to stop what you are doing to practise them. You can do them while you are washing up, watching TV or waiting for a bus. No one will know! The more often you can do them, the quicker you will see an improvement in the control you have over your bladder or bowel.

Taking care of yourself

There are a number of things you can do that may help to reduce incontinence and make life easier and more comfortable for yourself. It is really a question of getting to know your own body and your personal needs, as outlined in this section.

Do you go to the toilet regularly enough (about every two to three hours during the daytime)? You could use an alarm clock to remind yourself if necessary.

If you are taking diuretic drugs, which are usually prescribed to be taken in the morning, you will have to go to the toilet much more frequently — about half an hour after taking the drug and then hourly until lunch time.

Is the toilet well-lit and warm? Are there grab rails to help you up or down if you need them? Could clothes be made easier to unfasten or remove? What about velcro-fastened clothes or specially designed underwear? (See page 52 for more information about special clothing.)

Is your bed firm, easy to get out of and near enough to the toilet? Would a commode or urinal make night-times more comfortable? What about a waterproof mattress cover? There is a wide variety of waterproof bedding protection (see also page 53).

Do your clothes smell? You can avoid the risk of smelling by washing any clothing or bedding as soon as it becomes wet. If you want to leave clothing until you have a full load for the washing machine, rinse it straight away and leave it to soak. Don't leave anything to soak for longer than about 24 hours, and do not leave anything that is wet with urine to dry, as this will make it smell. Avoid washing powders with biological enzymes which may cause skin irritation when clothing becomes wet with urine.

Having a daily bath or body wash will give you the confidence that you smell fresh and encourage you to enjoy normal intimate contact with family and friends. You do not need to use disinfectants or antiseptics — these can kill off the useful bacteria that help to keep skin healthy. For men with urinary incontinence there is often a problem of smell. There are preparations available from chemists which can be applied to underpants to prevent smell and give you a feeling of confidence. Use perfumed products with care, as they can irritate sensitive skin.

Is incontinence affecting your sex life? There is no reason why your condition should prevent you having a satisfying sex life with your partner. Bathing before intercourse will help you feel confident and fresh. If you have a bladder problem, emptying your bladder just before intercourse may help to prevent leakage. (Some women find that the 'on top' position reduces the risk of leakage, as it puts less stress on the bladder and the pelvic floor muscles.) If you have a bowel problem, you can be fairly sure that once the bowel has emptied, there is unlikely to be another bowel movement for several hours, unless there is diarrhoea. One or two towels underneath you may help you feel more confident and comfortable in case of leakage.

Incontinence does not normally cause any pain during intercourse. If you feel any pain you should see your health adviser. Incontinence is not 'catching' in any way, so there is no medical reason why you and your partner should not enjoy full intercourse. But if either of you find the thought offputting, it is worth discussing your feelings with a sex therapist, who may be able to help you both find other ways of achieving sexual fulfilment. Also very useful is the book *Living, Loving and Ageing*, published by Age Concern (see page 77 for more details).

Treatment to cure or manage incontinence

If your problem is severe or has been going on for a long time, you will probably need some form of treatment in addition to self-help methods. This section describes some of the common forms of treatment. Your health adviser will help you decide which is most appropriate for your needs — including special exercises, re-training your bladder, medication and, in a few cases, surgery.

Doing exercises

If your problem is stress incontinence, the exercises described on page 40 to strengthen the pelvic floor muscles will probably be one of the first suggestions.

Retraining your bladder

This is a technique to help you lengthen the time between visits to the toilet by developing control over your bladder. When you feel you want to pass water urgently, you practise holding on — at first just for a minute, building up to five or ten minutes, or even longer. This technique is particularly helpful for people who suffer from urge incontinence.

It is important for you or the person you care for to go to the toilet regularly when practising this retraining technique. The health adviser will help to identify the best times of the day for you, using the record made of your visits to the toilet and the occasions when you were incontinent (see sample record on page 33). As control increases, you should try to use the toilet only at the agreed times, and to hold on in between these times.

Taking medicines

Sometimes treatment includes the use of medicines as a temporary solution to prevent unpleasant symptoms and to give other methods of treatment a chance to work. Here is a list of some of the more frequently used drugs (with brand names in brackets) and the conditions they are used to treat:

For urinary tract infections Ampicillin (Penbritin, Vidopen); Amoxycillin (Amoxil); Trimethoprim (Monotrim, Syraprim, Trimopan); Nitrofurantoin (Furadantin); Nalidixic Acid (Negram).

For female stress incontinence Dienoestrol cream (Hormofemin); Conjugated Oestrogens (Premerin).

For overflow incontinence Phenoxybenzamine (Dibenyline).

For underactive bladder Distigmine (Ubretid).

For urge incontinence Imipramine (Tofranil); Flaxovate Hydrochlorine (Urispas); Terodiline (Micturine).

Bulking agents for constipation Isphagula Husk (Fybogel, Isogel and Regulan); Sterculia (Normacol).

Laxatives Lactulose (Dulphalac); Danthron and Docusate (Co-Danthrusate, Normax); Sodium Picosulphate (Laxoberal, Picolax); Senna (Senokot).

Bladder infections You may be given drugs to help reduce the frequency of bladder contractions. These will also reduce the urgent need to pass water, but it is important at the same time to keep up a routine for bladder retraining or going to the toilet regularly. If you suffer from this condition and you are a woman who has passed the menopause, oestrogen creams or tablets are sometime effective. They help to reduce dryness and irritation of the vagina and urethra.

Overflow incontinence Drugs can be used to help your bladder contract properly and cause urine to flow from the bladder.

Stress or faecal incontinence caused by constipation You may be treated with one of the laxatives listed above or with suppositories or enemas. Many laxatives can be bought from the chemist without a prescription; but it is always advisable to seek medical advice first, as a laxative taken over long periods of time or in high doses can lead to a lazy bowel and a lack of some of the essential vitamins and minerals which our bodies require.

Using catheters

If you have an underactive bladder and are unable to empty it completely, you may need to use a catheter. This is a very thin tube which is inserted into the urethra and allows urine to drain from the bladder.

Self-catheterisation If your health adviser suggests using a catheter to empty your bladder at regular intervals, you will be shown how to insert and remove the catheter yourself. This may sound difficult to manage; but once you have become used to it, you will enjoy the flexibility it gives you. The health adviser will help you to decide how often and when you need to use it.

Long-term use of catheter Some bladder conditions are not suitable for treatment by intermittent use of a catheter. If it is impractical to use other methods — for example, because you are confined to bed — you may then need a catheter which is left in more permanently and which drains into a bag. The catheter will usually be left in for between two weeks and six months before being changed.

The long-term use of a catheter is only necessary in a few cases (about one in fifty). Your health adviser will want to avoid this if other solutions can be found.

Having surgery

In a few cases an operation may be needed to improve the condition. Talk to your doctor to find out whether your incontinence problem may be helped by surgery.

For women this is more likely when the pelvic muscles have stretched beyond improvement by exercise. A simple operation can be done to lift the neck of the bladder back into its former position where it was supported by the pelvic floor muscles. An operation usually means spending about a week in hospital and taking things easy for about six weeks afterwards. Immediately after surgery you will have a catheter inserted to empty your bladder. This will stay in place for two or three days until your bladder is working normally. You will need to do regular exercises to prevent the pelvic muscles weakening again.

For men the problem which is most likely to need surgery is an enlarged prostate gland. This can block the flow of urine from the bladder. The gland can be removed in a simple operation which normally means spending four or five days in hospital. After the operation you will have a catheter for two or three days to drain urine into a bag. Having your prostate gland removed will not make you impotent. It may affect ejaculation, in that sometimes sperm and seminal fluid pass into the bladder instead of through the tip of the penis. This is not harmful or painful and the fluid passes out through the urethra next time you urinate.

After both these operations you need to take things easy for three or four weeks. It is wise to avoid strenuous exercise such as digging and lifting heavy weights for around four to six weeks or until you feel fully fit again. Both men and women can enjoy an active sex life after these operations once they are fully recovered. If you have any doubts about this, talk to your health adviser.

Products, Services and Financial Help

This chapter outlines the wide range of equipment and products available to help cope with incontinence. The items may be obtainable on prescription (eg catheters); supplied free depending on where you live (eg incontinence pads); available for loan (eg commodes, bedpans); or available for purchase (eg special clothing). There are also points to consider when choosing what is right for your needs. The professionals who may be able to help or advise about products and local services provided by the council and health authority are also explained.

In addition the chapter describes some sources of financial help which may be available to people (including carers) who are coping with incontinence.

Choosing products with professional help

You should get professional advice in choosing a product to suit your condition (or that of the person you care for). Some products are designed specifically for men or women. With others, men and women need to learn different techniques to use them. Your choice will also be affected by individual needs and circumstances. You need to feel comfortable about using a particular article. If your problem is recent, the health adviser will help you choose the device or products that are right for you.

After using a product for some time, you will need to see your health adviser again to check whether it is still suitable or the best option for you. New and improved products are being developed all the time, and there may be something better than the one you are currently using. Your condition may also change and require something different to help you manage it. Other people who may also offer advice or practical help with products, equipment or services are listed on page 55.

Here are some points to consider before you consult a health adviser about choosing products or equipment. Bear in mind that you may need more than one item to cope with different activities and at different times of day.

Points to consider:

Do you need protection during the day or at night? At home or when going out?

How active will you be when using the system — walking, standing, exercising, sitting, lying down? Is it sufficiently water-proof and comfortable in all positions?

Do you need extra protection for long periods of sitting or lying down?

Will the product cause skin irritation if used over a long period of time?

Is the article easy to change or empty? How often does it need changing? Is it disposable? Are spares easy to carry?

Do products vary in size and absorbency? Which would suit you most?

What is the cost involved? Is it available on prescription?

Is it easy to obtain regular supplies?

You may need to try out a product for a period of time before you can answer some of these questions. Use them to judge how successful a particular system is in meeting your needs. You may not find the perfect answer straight away — it is more a matter of trying out a number of items until you find the one (or a combination) that you are happiest with.

Choosing products to wear

Looking after you skin

This is important if you have to wear a pad or other type of product next to your skin. Washing with mild soap and water should help to keep your skin healthy. It is a good idea to wash each time you change a pad or device if you can, but your health adviser will guide you on this. Creams, lotions and powders are not usually necessary and may increase the risk of skin problems by keeping the skin too wet or too dry.

Pad and pant systems

Pad and pant systems come in many different shapes and sizes which provide varying levels of absorbency. They can be used by both men and women by adjusting the position of the pad so that it gives maximum absorbency. Alternative solutions for men with bladder control problems may be more effective and are described at the end of this section.

There are a number of pad and pant systems to choose from, and these are described below. In some areas, pads can be obtained free through the continence adviser or GP, though the range is often limited. In other areas, free pads are supplied only to people who are severely incontinent. Your health adviser will be able to tell you what is available in your area.

Stretch pants with pads The pads for this type of system are waterproof backed and are usually rectangular or shaped to fit comfortably between the legs. The pads come in a wide range of sizes and levels of absorbency. They can be worn with your usual underpants — provided they are close-fitting — but they are more effective when worn with special stretch pants, as illustrated. Some pads have a piece of adhesive tape on their backing which sticks to the pants and gives extra security when you move about.

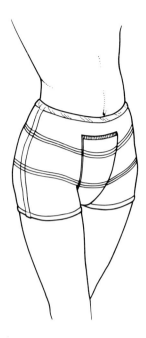

Advantages — flexible system, variety of fittings and types, pads not too bulky, easy to dispose of and to carry spares. Some pads with good width at back suitable for faecal incontinence.

Disadvantages — not really suitable for severe incontinence.

Pad worn with pants with a pouch Special pants with a waterproof pouch hold a pad firmly in position. You can slip the pad into the pouch from the outside or in some cases the inside of the pants. Your skin is protected from contact with the pad by a one-way liner which usually remains dry.

Advantages — pad is securely held, skin may be protected from constant contact with urine.

Disadvantages — only suitable for light to moderate urinary incontinence, messy to remove pads from pouch. Not suitable for faecal incontinence.

All-in-one pad and pant system These are available in both disposable and re-usable forms. They are similar to disposable nappies and come in a range of adult sizes. They may be useful to use at home at night, but should be combined with another system during the day or while going out.

Advantages — highly absorbent, suitable for heavy urinary incontinence, disposable type suitable for faecal incontinence.

Disadvantages — bulky to wear, dispose of and carry around. Expensive.

Absorbent pants These are similar to ordinary underpants, and they are made in washable fabric (most styles can be machine washed). The gusset has a waterproof backing which stops small amounts of urine from leaking through. A good fit is important with this type of pant — there is a good range of sizes, styles and colours to choose from.

Advantages — neat-fitting, washable.

Disadvantages — only suitable for light urinary incontinence.

Disposable pants These can be useful when away from home or when washing facilities are limited. They are suitable for faecal incontinence (unless there is diarrhoea) or can be used with a waterproof backed pad for urinary incontinence.

Advantages — totally disposable.

Disadvantages — expensive, making them unsuitable for long-term use.

Plastic pants Usually these are used with wadding cut to size off a roll. This system is cheap, suitable for urinary and faecal incontinence but is not a particularly comfortable choice.

Advantages — cheapest system, thickness of wadding can be varied to give more or less absorbency.

Disadvantages — plastic can cause a lot of sweating and chapping, is noisy and uncomfortable to wear.

Considerations for men Although most pant and pad systems are suitable for both men and women, some systems will provide greater protection against leakage if the position of the pad is adjusted. Men wearing a pad with stretch fabric pants or pants with a pouch need to place the pad more to the front to give maximum absorbency there. The pad needs to be at least 4 inches wide to give good widthways protection as well.

Choose a system which allows you to use the lavatory easily when you need to. Pants with fly openings are available so that you don't have to pull down your trousers.

Collection devices for men

These are another option for men who have problems with bladder control and may provide a better solution than using a pant and pad system. You could use a sheath system or a body-worn urinal both of which are connected with a tube to a drainage bag. Or you might find a drip collector gives you sufficient protection if you only suffer from slight leakage. There is quite a wide range of products with a variety of features to suit different levels of incontinence.

Sheath system This consists of a sheath made of lightweight latex which is attached to the penis by a special adhesive or a strap. The sheath has a tube, the lower end of which is connected

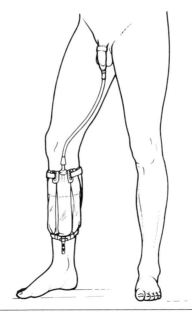

up to a drainage bag attached to the leg. One advantage of using a sheath is that it does not need to be fitted by an expert. It can be used for a day or two and then replaced. Sheaths are particularly suitable if you only need protection at certain times.

Body worn urinals These are collection devices made from latex rubber which fit over the penis. They are held in place by straps around the hips and the urine drains into a legbag. Body worn urinals need an experienced fitter to help choose a type and size which is comfortable for the wearer.

Drip collectors These are pouches made of disposable or re-usable material which fit over the penis. They are held in place by a strap around the hips or in some cases by well fitting pants. They are designed to collect only small quantities of urine.

Drainage bags

There are several types which can be used with male collection devices and with catheters by both men and women. For daytime use, there are small bags which are attached directly to the leg with straps or held in place inside a cloth bag. For the night, you can fix a larger bag to your leg so that you will not be disturbed during your sleep by the need to change it. Night drainage bags can also be attached to a bed-side holder or taped to your bed.

Clothes

If you find it hard to undo buttons and zips, there is underwear which fastens at the side and can be opened without having to be pulled down. Pants are made in a number of different styles, sizes and colours for men and women.

It may be possible to adapt your existing clothes to help you to undress more quickly by using velcro fastening and elasticated waists. Open-crotch pants and tights or wrap-around skirts with a large overlap at the back are suggestions for women. Trousers with velcro fastening may be useful for men.

For more detailed information about adapting clothes, contact the Disabled Living Foundation (see 'Helpful Organisations').

Choosing equipment

Bed protection

If you are likely to have any leakage from your bladder or bowels during the night, having your bed well protected will make for a peaceful night's sleep. A range of products is available, as outlined below.

Waterproof mattress covers These come in various sizes, but semi-fitted or fitted types are easiest.

Bedding covers These come in waterproof breathable material to go over pillows, duvets and blankets.

Absorbent sheets There are disposable and re-usable ones to help keep the skin dry.

Absorbent bed pads Most of these are re-usable, have a waterproof backing and are designed to be laid on directly or to be used under a one-way absorbent sheet. These pads help keep you dry and comfortable during the night, so be sure to wear night clothes that will not get in the way and be soaked by urine.

Bed alarms These work by setting off a bleeper or humming tone when a specially designed bed pad becomes wet. The alarms are run on batteries and may be useful if you, or your carer, need to wake when the bed has become wet.

Commodes, bedpans, hand-held urinals

For items such as chemical toilets, commodes and bedpans, your local health authority or social services department may have a loan service. Health authorities usually only lend equipment for up to three months, but social services departments can arrange long-term loans. If you are confined to bed or your toilet is some distance from your bedroom or living area, one of these aids may be what you need. Ask the doctor, district nurse, or local social services office about loan services in your area.

Hand-held 'slipper' urinal These are particularly useful for using at night, as the shaped end can be slipped under your bottom, and there is no need to sit on the urinal, as with a bedpan. If you need to use a urinal more than once during the night, keep a commode or bucket near the bed.

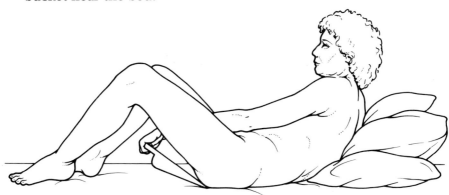

Buying or borrowing equipment and supplies

Large chemists stock supplies such as pad and pant systems, and waterproof bedding covers. They will often give advice about choosing products as well.

There are differences in what equipment or supplies each health authority will provide free of charge or on loan. Your local continence adviser or the district health service will be able to give information on this and on the range of products available.

There are Disabled Living Centres in most regions which have a wide range of aids and equipment on display. If you are near one, it may be worthwhile paying a visit (see 'Helpful Organisations' on page 68).

You may be able to borrow equipment from your local social services department (in the phone book under the name of the local council), or from the British Red Cross, St John Ambulance, Women's Royal Voluntary Service or some Age Concern groups (see 'Helpful Organisations').

Other professional help

There are other professionals who may be able to give help and advice. Ask your GP or continence adviser how to get in touch.

Social worker Gives advice about financial and practical help available through the local social services department. You may be entitled to a special laundry service, or be able to have grab rails or a raised seat put in to help you use your toilet. Equipment such as a commode is often available on loan. Contact by phoning your local social services office.

Occupational therapist Can advise about equipment, clothing and adaptations to your home if they are necessary. Contact through your local social services office.

Physiotherapist Can help to improve your mobility if this is a problem, using massage and special exercises. An obstetric physiotherapist can explain pelvic floor exercises. Usually hospital based, 'physios' may be contacted through the GP.

Local services

Help in the home Contact your local social services department, Age Concern group or Citizens Advice Bureau (in the phone book) to find out what help local organisations can offer in the home. Services such as meals-on-wheels, home helps or home care assistants may be available free or for a charge, depending on your income. Social services should also be able to advise about aids and adaptations in the home — for example, grab rails to make using the toilet easier. The Age Concern Fact Sheet *Finding help at home* provides further detailed information (see 'Information Factsheets' page 80.)

Laundry services Your local social services department or health authority may provide a laundry service. In some areas there is no laundry service available, but help at home with laundry may be given through the home care assistant service.

Laundry services are usually for bed linen and sometimes clothing, and offer a collection and delivery service. There is usually a small charge. To find out whether there is a laundry service in your area, ask your social worker, district nurse, GP or continence adviser, or contact your social services department or district health authority.

Disposal of waste Soiled incontinence pads should be wrapped in a plastic bag. They can be put in the dustbin or bin bag along with ordinary household rubbish for collection by the normal refuse disposal service. In some areas the council refuse department or the health authority provide special disposal bags and collection services for used incontinence pads. Phone your council refuse department or ask your GP, district nurse or continence adviser for more information.

Special help for disabled people

The local authority is legally bound to assess your special requirements for aids or an adaptation to your home and provide necessary services. In practice, however, the laws (Chronically Sick and Disabled Person's Act 1970 and the Disabled Person's Act 1986) leave it up to each local authority to decide how it will meet the needs of disabled people and how much care will be available.

The NHS and Community Care Act 1990 includes a requirement for local and health authorities to develop plans to show how they will meet the care needs of people living in their communities. Local authorities will also be given responsibility for people's need for community care services.

In carrying out these assessments, they will be required to co-operate with other authorities such as those for health and housing. However, now and in the future, it is left to each authority to decide what kinds of services to provide and how much of any service will be available. If help for incontinence sufferers is being cut back in your area, you might like to seek help from your local councillor, the community health council or your MP.

Some financial benefits

Although the Social Security System seems confusing, it is worth making the effort to claim what you are entitled to for yourself or the person you are caring for. The leaflets and claim forms mentioned in this section are available from the local social security office (in the phone book under 'Social Security' or 'Health and Social Security').

For a comprehensive guide to money benefits for older people, you may also want to read *Your Rights*, published by Age Concern (see page 77 for details).

Attendance allowance

This is a benefit for severely disabled people who need assistance or supervision with their personal needs, including help with bodily functions such as washing or using the toilet. It does not depend on your National Insurance contributions, is not affected by savings or income, and will not normally affect other benefits or pensions you receive. (But Attendance Allowance is counted as income when you apply for Income Support to help pay for residential or nursing home care).

You can receive the allowance if you live alone — what matters is that you need a high level of personal care, not that you are actually getting it. There are two rates: the lower one where night *or* daytime attention is needed, and the higher one where night *and* daytime attention is needed.

When you apply, a doctor will arrange to visit and make a report. Before the doctor's visit, it is a good idea to make a list of the help you need. Write down all the daily needs and tasks which you need help with. If you find a task particularly tiring, or can only do some things very slowly, mention this. Add anything else that you think may be relevant, such as how often or how many times help is needed during the night.

More information Leaflet NI 205 explains who is eligible and how to claim the Allowance, and includes an application form. Also do note that the Government has announced that it plans changes to the Attendance

Allowance which may be introduced in 1992, but these will only apply to people disabled before the age of 65.

Invalid care allowance (ICA)

This is a benefit paid to people under pension age who are unable to work full time because they spend 35 hours or more per week looking after someone who receives or is entitled to Attendance Allowance. You will not be able to get ICA if your earnings are over a certain level and may not receive any extra money if you are already receiving another social security benefit or your spouse is receiving an increase in his or her benefit for you.

Invalid Care Allowance is counted as income when assessing whether you are eligible for Income Support, Housing Benefit or Community Charge Benefit. But from October 1990 you may be entitled to a higher level of benefit, as the Government is introducing a Carer's Premium for some carers on a low income.

More information Leaflet NI 212 explains who is eligible and how to claim, and includes an application form.

The Social Fund

This provides lump-sum payments to people on low incomes to help cover the cost of large items that could not be met out of the weekly income. Normally, to get help from the Social Fund you need to be receiving Income Support and have limited savings. If you have difficulty with exceptional expenses due to in-continence (for example, replacing bedding or buying special equipment), you may qualify for help. Payments are made in the form of a budgeting loan, crisis loan, or community care grant, at the discretion of Social Fund Officers.

More information Leaflet SB 16 explains who may be eligible for help from the Social Fund and the different types of payment that are made. Ask for application form SF 300 to apply for a budgeting loan or community care grant. Ask immediately at the Social Security office if you need a crisis loan. It is worth getting help with your application from a welfare rights agency or Citizens Advice Bureau.

Independent Living Fund

This fund is to assist severely disabled people on low incomes who need to buy in help with personal care or domestic duties to enable them to remain living at home. It is for people who receive the higher rate of Attendance Allowance and mainly for people who live alone; but payment may sometimes be considered where a disabled person lives with a carer who is unable to fulfil all the tasks involved in caring. Do note that for the foreseeable future someone aged 75 or more is not eligible.

More information Details and an application form can be obtained from the Independent Living Fund, PO Box 183, Nottingham NG8 3RD. Telephone 0602 290427. Also note that the Fund was set up for a maximum of five years, so after 1993 there may be changes in the help available.

Help in Residential or Nursing Homes

The first part of this chapter is for care staff who are looking after someone with an incontinence problem in a communal setting — in a residential or nursing home. It gives additional information and advice on attitudes to incontinence; assessment; environmental factors; and practical help, guidance and training available to paid carers.

The second part of the chapter is for relatives and friends of people being cared for in a residential or nursing home. It gives information and advice on practical help that may be available; finding out about the daily routine and toilet facilities; and what to do if you are not satisfied with the help available for incontinent residents.

Practical support for care assistants

Some of the suggestions in this section are relevant to managers, others are more relevant to staff involved in the day-to-day physical care of residents. Statistics show that the highest figures for incontinence in older people are for those living in hospitals, private residential homes and nursing homes. Some aspects of living in an institutional setting increase the likelihood of becoming incontinent. Some older people in communal settings may be severely affected by conditions such as mental infirmity and mobility problems.

Care staff have a key role to play in helping older people to live with dignity and in encouraging each individual, whatever their circumstances, to achieve and maintain as much independence and control over their own situation as they are able to.

Attitudes to incontinence

Incontinence can have a devastating effect on the life of the person suffering from it, who may experience a loss of confidence and self-respect, and even feelings of disgust. As discussed on pages 27-29, some individuals may even deny that there is a problem because the truth is too painful to accept. As a carer, you are in a unique position to help overcome these feelings — but only if you are clear about your own attitudes to incontinence. It is not pleasant mopping up after someone, and you should try not to let the unpleasant aspects of coping with incontinence influence the way you treat the person.

Having a well-thought-out policy on how the Home handles incontinence and making use of all the practical help available can greatly reduce the work involved in helping someone to manage their incontinence. For example, both managers and care staff need to agree and co-operate in managing daily routines such as going to the toilet so that these fit in with the needs of individual residents, rather than residents being required to fit in with routines. Night staff also need to agree guidelines about whether and when to get residents up in the night.

If you are a manager, consider developing a policy and practical guidelines, if these do not exist, in consultation with staff. If you are responsible for the practical care of residents, you could consider asking your manager or supervisor whether it would be possible to develop such guidelines.

Assessment

Any resident who has a bladder or bowel problem should have their condition assessed regularly. This will require a co-ordinated approach on the part of staff in the Home. It may need the involvement of the person's GP or the continence adviser. It may sometimes seem easier simply to 'cope' with incontinence, but the time involved in arranging a proper assessment can be well worthwhile — provided it helps the resident feel less anxious and makes the situation easier to manage for staff. Managers and care staff may find it helpful to discuss together the following suggest-ions for action.

▶ Get a history of the resident's continence/incontinence and health.

▶ Keep a record to establish the pattern and type of incontinence.

▶ Refer the resident to the GP so that tests can be done to discover any physical or psychological causes of the problem.

▶ Make any changes to the environment necessary to help regain continence.

▶ Make sure the resident is not cutting down on liquids; but if there is night-time incontinence, try giving the last drink earlier in the evening to see whether this helps, as suggested in the chapter 'Regaining Control'.

▶ Draw up a care plan with the resident and other staff — this may include pelvic floor exercises, routines for going to the toilet or bladder retraining (also covered in 'Regaining Control'), or the use of continence products and equipment.

▶ Ask for the help of the continence adviser if the aims of the care plan are not achieved. (If there is no continence adviser for your area, your Home might press for one to be appointed.)

▶ If it is not possible for the resident to become fully continent, the aim of the care plan should be to help the person manage effectively, comfortably and as independently as possible.

Environment

The physical surroundings in which older people live can have a profound effect on whether they remain continent or not. In particular it is essential for an older person to have easy access to a toilet at all times. Here are some questions to ask yourself about the toilet facilities in the home where you work:

▶ Are there enough toilets? (At least one to every four residents?)

- ▶ Are they easy to get to? at night? during the day? As shown in the drawing on page 64 the toilet should be no further than 20 metres from sitting room, dayroom or bedroom areas.
- ▶ Are they comfortable? well-lit? well-heated? with washing and disposal facilities?
- ▶ Is the height of the seat comfortable? Are there grab-rails?
- ▶ Can residents get help when they want to use the toilet with a walking aid or from a helper?
- ▶ If residents have difficulties getting to the toilet, are commodes or urinals available?
- ▶ Is help always provided in a sensitive way with the aim of maintaining dignity and, as far as possible, privacy?

If there are fixed or routine times for visits to the toilet, check that these fit in with the individual's needs. Keeping a record of visits to the lavatory or accidents that have occurred can sometimes pinpoint times which are 'high risk'. It may be possible to avoid accidents by simply bringing forward a visit to the toilet or by providing help to get there.

Motivation

If the daily routine makes it difficult for residents to get to the toilet when they need to, or if people are left alone or allowed to become bored for long periods of time, the chances are that incontinence will increase. Rightly or wrongly, individuals may feel that wetting or soiling themselves is a way of gaining attention that they do not otherwise receive. If residents are left sitting on commodes, or are padded up all the time, this removes both their dignity and the motivation to try and maintain control of their condition.

The organisation of routines, the available facilities, the level of stimulus in daily interests and activities and the care and sensitivity of staff all contribute to an environment and atmosphere which may either encourage or discourage continence.

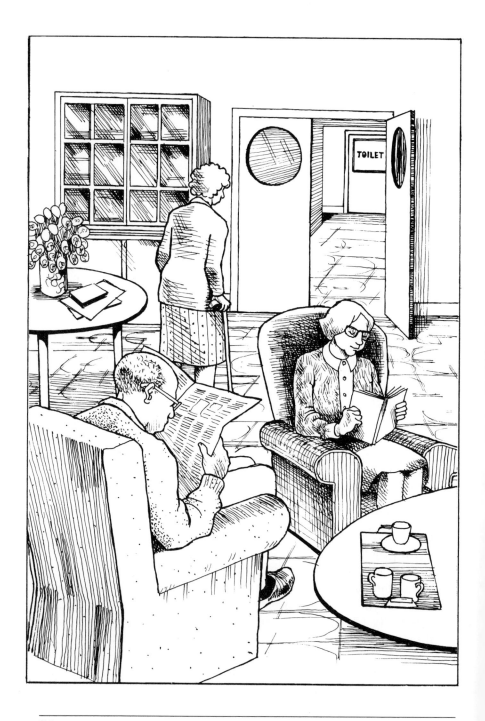

Practical help

It is worth checking what practical help is available to the residential or nursing home you work in from the district health service and from your local social services department. Policies of health and local authorities are all different, but some assistance in the form of loan of equipment, special collection service for used pads and other products is usually offered. Your local continence adviser will be able to give you more information.

Guidance and training for paid carers

Continence advisers offer guidance and often training on the management of continence to paid carers within their area. You may also be able to borrow videos or self-study materials on managing continence, like those produced by the training department at Age Concern England.

The Disabled Living Foundation and some other organisations hold study days on promoting continence. The English National Board for Nursing, Health Visiting and Midwifery has developed a short course which runs at various centres around the country, and similar courses are run in other regions in the UK. Health Education Units can also provide written information and advice.

Taking Good Care is a practical book for care assistants and other carers covering all aspects of the caring process also published by Age Concern (see 'Useful Publications' on page 72 for details).

Practical support for residents

This section offers advice for relatives and friends of a resident about practical aspects of the care provided and support that may be available from sources outside the Home or hospital.

Practical and financial help

Anyone living in a residential home should be entitled to the same help with incontinence as someone who lives in their own home. Some health authorities will help people in local authority homes but not in private ones. Some residential homes charge for incontinence supplies as 'extras', but you could check whether these supplies are available through the NHS by seeking advice from your local Community Health Council. Someone living in a nursing home may be charged extra for incontinence aids,depending on the home.

The community nurse or continence adviser for the area may be able to give advice or visit a resident to assess their needs, though this service varies between health authorities. Sometimes a charge is made for a continence adviser to visit a private home.

Daily routines and toilet facilites

Several studies have shown that changes in the daily routine can help to increase continence in older people living in a communal setting. It is important to find out from residents whether there are enough toilets, and whether people are helped if necessary to go to the toilet at regular intervals, rather than just at mealtimes. It is worth checking that clothing can be unfastened easily, and that people are not just 'padded up' rather than being helped to manage their continence.

Aspects of the wider environment mentioned on page 62 can also affect whether people feel motivated to manage their incontinence in a communal setting. The attitude of staff and the atmosphere of the Home should encourage, but can in some cases inadvertently discourage continence.

Improving the help available

If someone with incontinence is not receiving the care and practical help that they need, there is a risk that their condition will get worse. It is naturally in the interests of both residents and staff to help someone with a bladder or bowel problem to manage as independently as they can. If, as a relative or friend, you are not satisfied with the help that is given, you could:

▶ Tactfully talk about your concerns to the person in charge of the Home.

▶ Ask for the community nurse or continence adviser to visit and advise.

▶ If no help is forthcoming, take up matters with the registration officer of the social services department, or in the case of a nursing home, with the health authority registration officer. (Contact them through the local social services office or district health authority headquarters.) The registration officers may be able to take up the matter with the manager or proprietor of the Home.

If several people are concerned about this issue, you could together consider pressing the health authority to appoint a continence adviser where there is none or to provide free incontinence supplies. This can sometimes produce results. Your Community Health Council or local Age Concern may be able to give advice on how to go about this.

Resources and Information

Helpful Organisations

The organisations listed here may be able to give information, help or advice in a variety of different ways, but this is not an exhaustive list. Most are national organisations, but some may have a local branch in your area (for information contact the national headquarters or look in your phone book). Your local library, Citizens Advice Bureau or local Age Concern may also be able to put you in touch with other helpful organisations.

Alzheimer's Disease Society

For carers of people with any form of dementia, details of local groups and a guide on caring for someone with dementia.

158-160 Balham High Road
London SW12 9BN
Tel: 081-675 6557

Association of Continence Advisors

For information about where to contact a local continence adviser.

Disabled Living Foundation
380-384 Harrow Road
London W9 2HU
Tel: 071-266 3704

British Red Cross

For details of local branches for free short-term loan of commodes, urinals and other equipment.

Main Headquarters
9 Grosvenor Crescent
London SW1X 7EJ
Tel: 071-235 5454

Carers National Association

Support, information and local groups for people caring for someone at home.

29 Chilworth Mews
London W2 3RG
Tel: 071-724 7776

Continence Advisory Service

Has information leaflets and advises on special clothing, aids and equipment.

Disabled Living Foundation
380-384 Harrow Road
London W9 2HU
Tel: 071-266 2059

Dene Centre

Continence Advisory Service for the North of England, offers advice and information leaflets.

Castles Farm Road
Newcastle-u-Tyne NE3 1PH
Tel: 091-284 0480
(see also 'Telephone Helplines')

Disability Alliance

Campaigns for disabled people and publishes Disability Rights Handbook.

25 Denmark Street
London WC2H 8NJ
Tel: 071-240 0806

Disability Scotland

24-hour information service for people with disabilities.

Princes House
5 Shandwick Place
Edinburgh EH2 4RG
Tel: 031-229 8632

Disabled Living Centres Council

For details of local living centres which display information and products and have facilities for trying out different aids.

Disabled Living Foundation
380-384 Harrow Road
London W9 2HU
Tel: 071-266 2059

Health Education Units

For information leaflets and details of useful local organisations.

(see under District Health Authority in your phone book)

Help the Aged

General information service for older people and their carers.

16-18 St James's Walk
London EC1R 0BE
Tel: 071–253 0253
Freephone 0800 289404

Holiday Care Service

Advice on holidays, holiday helpers and travel arrangements for disabled and older people.

2 Old Bank Chambers
Station Road
Horley, Surrey RH6 9HW
Tel: 0293 774535

Northern Ireland Council on Disability

Information and leaflets for people with disabilities.

2 Annadale Avenue
Belfast BT7 3JR
Tel: 0232 491011

RADAR (Royal Association for Disability and Rehabilitation)

For information on hotels and holidays for people suffering from incontinence.

25 Mortimer Street
London W1N 8AB
Tel: 071-637 5400

SPOD (Association to Aid the Sexual and Personal Relationships of People with a Disability)

For help and counselling on intimate relationships including sexual problems and incontinence.

286 Camden Road
London N7 0BJ
Tel: 071-607 8851

St John Ambulance Brigade

For details of local branches who may be able to arrange loan of commodes and urinals.

Edwina Mountbatten House
63 York Street
London WC1H 1PS
Tel: 071-258 3456

WRVS (Women's Royal Voluntary Service)

For leaflet on adapting clothes for people who are incontinent; details of local branches who may offer a delivery service for incontinence supplies.

234-244 Stockwell Road
London SW9 9SP
Tel: 071-733 3388

Telephone Helplines

Some organisations, and companies selling incontinence products, have confidential telephone advice services which you may find helpful.

Bard Helpline 0800 591 783

12.30 pm - 4.30 pm Monday-Friday, answerphone (as European Linkline) at other times.
(No charge)

Coloplast Service 0800 622 124

9.00 am - 5.00 pm Monday-Friday, answerphone at other times.
(No charge)

Dial UK (Disablement Information and Advice Line) 0302 310123

(Charged at ordinary rate for a phone call)

Health Call 0898 600 835

Three-minute tape on incontinence.
(Charged at ordinary rate for phone call)

Health Line
Ask for tape 83 on incontinence.

081-681 3311 (Croydon) 4 pm - 8 pm only
0392 59191 (Exeter) 24-hour service
0482 29933 (Hull) 24-hour service
(Charged at ordinary rate for phone call)

Hollister InCare Helpline 0800 521 377

9.00 am - 5.30 pm Monday-Friday, answerphone at other times.
(No charge)

Incontinence Information Helpline 091-213 0050

2.00 pm - 7.00 pm weekdays for people living in northern England.
(Charged at ordinary rate for phone call)

Useful Publications

A number of useful books and leaflets are listed here. Your local library will be able to help you find them — if they don't have a particular book, they may be able to get it from another library. Bookshops will order a book for you if they don't have it in stock.

Association of Continence Advisers (1988) *Directory of Continence and Toileting Aids*. Available from Disabled Living Foundation, 380-384 Harrow Road, London, W9 2HU.

Blannin, J P and Fenely R C L (1984) *Incontinence: Patient Handbook No 18*. Available from Retail Services Department, Longman Group UK Ltd, Pinnacles, Harlow, Essex, CM19 5AA.

Disability Alliance, *Disability Rights Handbook* (updated annually). Available from Disability Alliance, 25 Denmark Street, London WC2 6NJ.

Gartley, C B (1985) *Managing Incontinence: A guide to living with loss of bladder control*. Available from Souvenir Press.

Kohner, N (1988) *Caring at Home: A handbook for people looking after people at home*. Available from the National Extension College, 18 Brooklands Avenue, Cambridge, CB2 2HN.

Mandelstam, D *Understanding Incontinence*. Available from Chapman and Hall.

Mitchell, L (1988). *The Magic of Movement*.Available from Age Concern England, 1268 London Road, London SW 16 4EJ.

RADAR, *Holidays for Disabled People* and *Holidays and Travel Abroad — a guide for disabled people*. Available from RADAR, 25 Mortimer Street, London W1N 8AB.

RADAR, *Motoring and Mobility for Disabled People*. Available from RADAR, 25 Mortimer Street, London W1N 8AB.

Worsley, J (1989) *Taking Good Care; A handbook for care assistants*. Available from Age Concern England, 1268 London Road, London SW16 4EJ.

Leaflets and Factsheets

To get the leaflets and factsheets listed below, write to the organisations which produce them.

Age Concern England, Factsheet 23, *Help with incontinence.* Send sae to Information and Policy Dept., 1268 London Road, London SW16 4EJ. See page 80 for other Age Concern factsheets.

Coloplast Foundation, *Advice for carers of incontinent adults; Regaining bladder control.* Available from the Coloplast Foundation, Peterborough Business Park, Cambs, PE2 0XF.

Continence Advisory Service. Produces leaflets about incontinence. Available from DLF (Sales), Book House, 45 East Hill, London SW18 2QZ. Titles include:

Adult bedwetting;

Bladder training;

Confused incontinent person at home;

Notes on incontinence;

Stress incontinence;

Penile sheaths;

Your prostate operation.

Council and Care for the Elderly, *What to look for in a private or voluntary home.* Available from Council and Care for the Elderly.

Medical Assist, *Is laughing not a laughing matter?* Available from Medical Assist Ltd, Commerce Way, Colchester, Essex, CO2 8HH.

Northern Regional Continence Advisory Service, *Financial benefits and services for people with problems of incontinence.* Available from Dene Centre, Castles Farm Road, Newcastle-upon-Tyne, NE3 1PH.

About Age Concern

This is one of a wide range of publications produced by Age Concern England which is also actively engaged in training, information provision, research and campaigning for retired people and those who work with them. It is a registered charity dependent on public support for the continuation of its work.

Age Concern England links closely with Age Concern centres in Scotland, Wales and Northern Ireland to form a network of over 1400 independent local UK groups. Assisted by an estimated 250,000 volunteers, they aim to improve the quality of life for older people and develop services appropriate to local needs and resources — advice and information, day care, visiting services, transport schemes, specialist facilities for physically and mentally frail older people.

In particular, through its Age Well programme, initiated jointly with the Health Education Authority, Age Concern England is actively involved in promoting a healthier old age.

Age Concern England
Astral House
1268 London Road
London SW16 4EJ
Tel: 081-679 8000

Age Concern Scotland
54A Fountainbridge
Edinburgh EH3 9PT
Tel: 031-228 5656

Age Concern Wales
4th Floor
1 Cathedral Road
Cardiff CF1 9SD
Tel: 0222 371821/371566

Age Concern Northern
Ireland
6 Lower Crescent
Belfast BT7 1NR
Tel: 0232 245729

Other Publications from Age Concern

A wide range of titles are available under the Age Concern imprint.

Health

Your Health in Retirement Dr J A Muir Gray and Pat Blair
A comprehensive guide to help people look after their health. Full details are given of health advisers and useful organisations to contact for help.

0-86242-082-2   £4.50

The Magic of Movement Laura Mitchell
Full of encouragement, this book by TV personality Laura Mitchell is for those who are finding everyday activities more difficult. Includes gentle exercises to tone up muscles and ideas to make you more independent and avoid boredom.

0-86242-076-8   £3.95

Know Your Medicines Pat Blair
This guide for older people and their carers explains how the body works and how it is affected by medication. Also included is guidance on using medicines and an index of commonly used medicines and their side effects.

0-86242-043-1   £3.95

The Foot Care Book: An A-Z of fitter feet Judith Kemp SRCh
A self-help guide for older people on routine foot care, this book includes an A-Z of problems, information on adapting and choosing shoes and a guide to who's who in foot care.

0-86242-066-0   £2.95

In Touch With Cateracts Margaret Ford
Over 20,000 cateract operations take place each year. Some patients have difficulties in adapting to their new vision. This booklet looks at ways of solving some of the problems and aims to allay anxieties.

0-86242-037-7   £1.00

Housing

Your Home in Retirement: An owner's guide Co-published with the NHTPC

This definitive guide considers all aspects of home maintenance of concern to retired people and those preparing for retirement, providing advice on heating, insulation and adaptations.

0-86242-095-4   £2.50

Housing Options for Older People David Bookbinder

A review of housing options is part of growing older. All the possibilities and their practical implications are carefully considered in this comprehensive guide.

0-86242-055-5   £2.50

Sharing Your Home Christine Orton

Guidelines for multi-generational families considering living together under the same roof. Includes information about the legal and financial factors as well as the emotional adjustments required.

0-86242-060-1   £1.95

A Buyer's Guide to Sheltered Housing Co-published with the NHTPC

Buying a flat or bungalow in a sheltered scheme? This guide provides vital information on the running costs, location, design and management of schemes to help you make an informed decision.

0-86242-063-6   £2.50

At Home In A Home Pat Young

The questions older people ask when considering moving into residential accommodation are answered in this practical guide. Such topics as fees, financial support and standards of care are tackled in realistic terms in order to help people make the right choice.

0-86242-062-8   £3.95

Money Matters

Your Rights 1990-91 Sally West

A highly acclaimed annual guide to the State benefits available to older people. Contains current information on retirement pensions, means-tested benefits as well as other financial help in paying for health and residential care, transport and legal fees.

0-86242-089-X   £1.95

Your Taxes and Savings 1990-91 John Burke, Joanna Hanks,
Simon Richmond
Explains how the tax system affects people over retirement age, includes
advice on independent taxation and how to avoid paying more tax than
necessary. The information about savings covers the wide range of
investment opportunities now available.

0-86242-093-8   £3.50

Using Your Home as Capital Cecil Hinton
This best selling book for home-owners, which is updated annually,
gives a detailed explanation of how to capitalise on the value of your
home and obtain a regular additional income.

0-86242-096-2   £2.95

General

Living, Loving and Ageing Wendy Greengross and Sally Greengross
Sexuality is often regarded as the preserve of the younger generation. At
last, here is a book for older people, and those who care for them, which
tackles the issues in a straightforward fashion, avoiding preconceptions
and bias.

0-86242-070-9   £4.95

Famous Ways to Grow Old Philip Bristow
A collection of letters from internationally distinguished people, outlin-
ing their personal attitudes to the onset of old age.

0-86242-087-3   £8.95

Survival guide for Widows June Hemer and Ann Stanyer
Widows describe what grieving has meant to them. Other people with
experience of the practical side of widowhood give guidance on Wills,
taxation, social security, housing and living alone.

0-86242-049-0   £3.50

What Every Woman Should Know About Retirement Edited by
Helen Franks
Retirement for women may appear less drastic a change than for men; but
it is, in many ways, more complex, affecting many parts of their lives.
These include marriage, living alone, financial planning, caring for
someone, looking after health and appearance.

0-86242-054-7   £4.50

Life in the Sun: A guide to long-stay holidays and living abroad in retirement Nancy Tuft
Every year millions of older people consider either taking long-stay holidays or moving abroad on a more permanent basis. This essential guide examines the pitfalls associated with such a move and tackles topics varying from pets to poll tax.

0-86242-085-7   £6.95

Professional

A Warden's Guide to Healthcare in Sheltered Housing Dr Anne Roberts
An invaluable guide for all wardens and care home proprietors on the health needs of older people and the best means of promoting better health for their residents.

0-86242-052-0   £6.50

Taking Good Care Jenyth Worsley
Examines all aspects of the caring process, whether the carer is an assistant in a Residential Home or looking after an elderly friend or relative at home.

0-86242-072-5   £6.95

Cooking for Elderly People Alan Stewart
Designed for use by anyone catering for groups of older people. This excellent manual contains over 120 thoroughly tested recipes.

0-86242-046-0   £17.50

The Law and Vulnerable Elderly People Edited by Sally Greengross
This report raises fundamental questions about the way society views and treats older people. The proposals put forward seek to enhance the self-determination and autonomy of vulnerable old people to ensure that they are better protected in the future.

0-86242-050-4   £6.50

Old Age Abuse Mervyn Eastman
This book looks at three main aspects of old age abuse; the setting, the victims and the solutions. The studies are based on the author's 14 years as a social work practitioner. He presents the frustrating dilemma facing those people who act in violence to those whom they may love and the tragic consequences of these actions.

0-86242-030-X   £5.00

To order books, send a cheque or money order to the address below; postage and packing is free. Cheques should be made out to Age Concern England. Credit card orders may be made on 081-679 8000.

Age Concern England
FREEPOST
1268 London Road
London SW16 4EJ

Continence Training

Age Concern England has prepared the four packs listed below to meet the need for easy-to-read training materials which can be used in a one-day course. Each pack includes background reading for the trainer, overhead acetates for teaching sessions, card games, quizzes and a suggested programme.

The four packs are:

Continence Training for Volunteers;

Continence Training for Carers in the Community;

Continence Training for Residential Home Care Staff;

Continence Training for Multidisciplinary Groups of Carers;

Price of each pack £30.00 (incl. p&p).

To order one or more of the packs, send a cheque or postal order to:

Training Department
Age Concern England
Astral House
1268 London Road
London SW16 4EJ

Information Factsheets

Age Concern England produces factsheets on a variety of subjects, one of which has been mentioned on page 73 of *In Control*. Among the 30 factsheets produced, the following titles may be of use to readers of this book:

Help with Heating. Factsheet 1

Dental Care in Retirement. Factsheet 5

Finding Help at Home. Factsheet 6

Local Authorities and Residential Care. Factsheet 10

Raising Income or Capital From Your Home. Factsheet 12

Older Home Owners: Sources of Financial Help with Repairs. Factsheet 13

Income Related Benefits: Income and Capital. Factsheet 16

Legal Arrangements for Managing Financial Affairs. Factsheet 22

Finding Residential and Nursing Home Accomodation. Factsheet 29

To order the factsheets:
Single copies are free on receipt of a 9" x 6" sae.

If you require a selection of factsheets or multiple copies, charges will be given on request.

A complete set of factsheets is available in a ring binder at the current cost of £24, which includes the first year's subscription. The current cost for an annual subscription for subsequent years is £10. There are different rates of subscription for people living abroad.

Factsheets are revised and updated throughout the year and membership of the subscription service will ensure that your information is always current.

Write to:
Information and Policy Department
Age Concern England
Astral House
1268 London Road
London SW16 4EJ

We hope you found this book useful. If so,
perhaps you would like to receive further
information about Age Concern or help us do
more for elderly people.

Dear Age Concern
Please send me the details I've ticked below:

other publications
☐

Age Concern special offers
☐

volunteer with a local group
☐

regular giving
☐

covenant
☐

legacy
☐

Meantime, here is a gift of

£ _____ PO/CHEQUE or VISA/ACCESS No _____

NAME (BLOCK CAPITALS) _____

SIGNATURE _____

ADDRESS _____

_____

_____ POSTCODE _____

Please pull out this page and send it to: **Age Concern** (DEPT IC2)
FREEPOST
Mitcham,
no stamp needed **Surrey CR4 9AS**

YOUR HEALTH
IN RETIREMENT

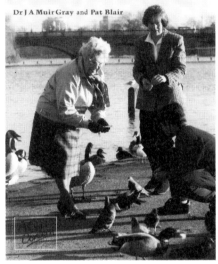

Dr J A Muir Gray and Pat Blair

£4.50

This book is a comprehensive source of information to help readers look after themselves and work towards better health. Produced in easy-to-read A–Z style, full details are given of people and useful organisations from which advice and assistance can be sought.

"full of helpful hints and information"
Woman & Home

ORDER FORM

Please send me .... copy/ies of **YOUR HEALTH in retirement.** I enclose a cheque/PO payable to Age Concern England for £............................

I authorise you to charge my Access/Visa card for £............................

The account number is

Card expiry date................Signature........................Date................
Credit card orders can also be made on 081-679 8000.
Name ....
Address ....
....
.... Postcode................

Please return this form, together with payment, to:
Department IC, Age Concern England, 1268 London Road, London, SW16 4EJ

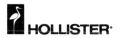

HOLLISTER®

AboutHollisterLimited

Products

The Hollister* InCare* Urinary Sheath

Designed to provide the wearer with optimum comfort and security, this technically advanced sheath remains securely in place, providing the wearer with a high level of efficient incontinence care that they can confidently rely on. A unique one-way flap prevents back flow of urine, keeping the penis comfortably dry and free from skin problems.

The Hollister* InCare* Leg Bag

Designed to the same high standard as the Urinary Sheath, this bag is held securely and comfortably in place even when full. It is simple to drain and can easily be adjusted by the wearer.

The Hollister* InCare* Faecal Collector

Clean, simple and convenient, this collector is designed to contain faeces and odour and only needs to be changed once in every 24 hours. Simple to fit and easy to change, the Faecal Collector also protects the user from skin soreness or irritation and is supremely comfortable to wear.

*Trademark of Hollister Incorporated USA

The Hollister InCare* Female Urinary Pouch*

Designed to provide a more efficient and dignified alternative to the use of absorbant pads, the Female Urinary Pouch is both highly convenient and comfortable. Leakproof and odour-free, the Female Urinary Pouch is nothing less than a revolution in female incontinence care.

Information, advice, problems?

Professional Services Team

This team is staffed by highly qualified professional advisors all of whom have had extensive experience in patient care. They will be pleased to provide confidential advice on any aspect of incontinence and the Hollister* InCare* range of Products as well as those of other manufacturers. Our Professional Services Team consists of the following people.

Jean Marceau The Manager of the team. A State Registered Nurse with many years experience, Jean was initially a Medical Ward Sister before working in Canada for two years and then a Surgical Ward Sister in a genito-urinary ward. Jean has received a Florence Nightingale award for her work as a Nursing Officer and brings nearly 15 years of experience in the UK and overseas to her position at Hollister Limited.

Auriol Lawson Previously a stoma care nurse and incontinence nurse at the Freeman Hospital, Newcastle, Auriol is a Clinical Specialist with many years experience. Although her main function is to develop educational services for specialised nurses and provide clinical support for our products, Auriol also assists us with our advisory service.

Anna Eagling Anna is our qualified Nurse Advisor who shares the responsibility with Jean in looking after telephone enquiries and letters from professionals and customers.

Confidential free advisory service

If you would like copies of fact sheets designed to explain the causes and treatment of urinary conditions associated with incontinence, please phone 0800 521377 or write to the address below.

Services

Customer Services Team

Our products are stocked by many chemists, but should you experience any difficulty in obtaining them, a member of our Customer Services Team will be pleased to help you. All orders are dealt with promptly and efficiently and are despatched by Securicor to guarantee delivery within 48 hours of your phone call or receipt of your prescription.

To order by Freephone dial 0800 521392

To order by post, write to:
Sales Service Department
Hollister Limited
43 Castle Street
Reading RG1 7SN